What to Expect as a Loved One's Death Draws Near

by Deborah Sigrist, B.S.N., R.N., CRNH

When my father's doctor told him he had three to six months to live, life was forever changed for our family. We began a journey full of unknowns and intense feelings. It felt like we were characters in a fairytale, setting out on a dangerous journey into an unknown land. How might we survive? What does it mean to "survive" this kind of a journey?

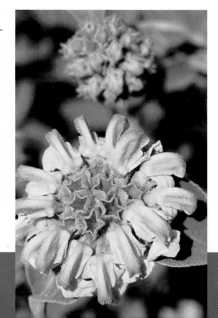

We needed landmarks, information, support, and courage. Perhaps you do, too.

Working your way through

No one can fully predict what to expect as you embark on this journey. No one is fully prepared to face every challenge. Here are some guidelines, however, that can help you cope at this difficult—and sacred—time.

■ *Re-frame how you see the dying process.*
Dying is a process that involves a slowing down, a breaking down, of the body. Often the change is gradual. At other times, however, deterioration can be quite rapid.

Dying is a unique process. How one dies often echoes how one has lived. For example, the stoic, private person is likely to approach death in that same way. Others will want to have many people around and may be quite expressive. We need to be cautious not to impose our own ideas of the "proper" way to die on someone else.

Dying involves the whole person, not just the body. Sometimes people feel emotionally and spiritually ready, but their bodies may not yet be ready. Other times the body may be racing towards death but the person is not yet ready to let go. Both the dying person and loved ones need much support in these situations.

A willingness to re-frame the dying process also includes expanding our understanding of the meaning of words such as *cure, healing*, and *hope*. An incurable illness is not "hopeless." Healing can occur whether or not a physical cure is possible. There are countless healings that can happen within oneself and one's relationships as death approaches. Seek out and nurture these healings.

■ *Understand the physical signs of dying.*

Dying is hard work. The body labors as it shuts down. This involves changes that at times can be troubling to witness, but are not usually medical emergencies. The changes are natural ways the body prepares itself for death. Measures that provide maximum comfort are the appropriate response.

A dying person's desire to eat diminishes. Food doesn't taste the same, eating becomes an effort; there may be nausea or vomiting. This is a difficult time for loved ones, because food sustains life and symbolizes love. Try to find out just what, when, and how much your loved one can comfortably eat. Trust that your loved one's body is taking the lead.

As eating and drinking taper off, the body becomes dehydrated. This is natural, and helps make the dying person sleepier and less aware of discomforts. Force feeding a body that can't handle it will cause serious complications. Sips of fluid, ice chips, and mouth swabbing can maintain comfort.

As the body weakens and slows down, fluid may build up in the lungs or the back of the throat. Breathing may sound moist or rattle-like. Secretions can best be managed with medications, regular turning and positioning, and the

It's important to remember that throughout the journey toward death, comfort can be maintained. Hospice caregivers specialize in assuring maximum comfort in response to the symptoms that accompany dying. Such holistic care emphasizes symptom management and quality of life. Comfort for the dying person and support for loved ones are hallmarks of hospice care, so be sure to take advantage of this option.

natural process of dehydration. Turning your loved one in bed every two to three hours is essential for preventing fluids from pooling in one area of the lungs. It's also important to protect the skin from pressure sores. Suctioning the throat or lungs is minimally useful and often uncomfortable for the dying person.

You matter to the last moment of your life, and we will do all we can, not only to help you die peacefully, but to live until you die.

—Dame Cicely Saunders
Founder, modern hospice movement

Because the kidneys and bowels are also shutting down, you can expect that urine output will gradually lessen and become more concentrated. A catheter may be needed to protect skin and prevent injury caused by climbing out of bed to get to the bathroom. Bowel movements become less frequent but still should be monitored because constipation can be uncomfortable. Most people lose control of bowel and bladder as muscles in that area begin to relax. One needs to keep the person clean and dry, especially to prevent skin breakdown.

As the body's senses tone down, vision may be blurred and communication more limited. Always assume the person can hear, though possibly not respond. A soothing environment and gentle touch are wonderful ways to communicate. In the words of Sister Betty Hopf, chaplain at St. Joseph's Regional Medical Center in South Bend, Indiana, "Touch is the ideal way to communicate with someone who may have trouble communicating. It's the first sense we experience when we're born, and—for the fortunate—the last one we experience when we die."

As the dying person nears the end of the journey, the body's most vital organs show signs of failure. As the heart can no longer do its job, the body conserves blood flow for the core organs. Blood then pools in the extremities, causing color and temperature changes. Hands, feet, and legs feel cool or cold to the touch. Fingers, nail beds, earlobes may look light gray or blue. Mottling, a blotchy purple skin tone, often appears on the knees and/or feet. The person may have a fever or the skin may feel cool and clammy. Avoid putting too many blankets on a person at this time.

Changes occur in breathing rate, depth, and rhythm. There may be periods of no breathing. The dying person doesn't experience this as suffocating, and is usually unconscious at this point. Blood pressure is very low by now and heart rate is rapid but weak. The body is clearly ready to be released.

■ *Prepare for mental and emotional changes.* Mental changes as death approaches may include confusion, restlessness, and agitation. This can be due to a

The experience of dying frequently includes glimpses of another world and those waiting in it. Although they provide few details, dying people speak with awe and wonder of the presence of people whom we cannot see —perhaps people they have known and loved. They know, often without being told, that they are dying, and may even tell us when their deaths will occur.
—Maggie Callanan and
Patricia Kelley
Final Gifts

variety of causes, including the disease itself, medications, metabolic changes, and lessened blood-flow to the brain. You can help by maintaining a soothing environment. Avoid over-stimulation; don't permit too many people in the room at one time. Provide an atmosphere in which your loved one feels safe and calm. If need be, medications can be adjusted or new ones introduced to provide rest.

The level of consciousness may range from alert and aware to deep coma. As death nears, don't be surprised if your loved one is asleep more than awake. Continue to assume your words are heard, however, and your presence felt.

Emotional changes vary with the person. Hopefully, feelings of fear, anxiety, regret, and concern have been discussed and expressed before mental clouding occurs, but don't force anything. It may be important for you, however, to find ways to say goodbye.

It's normal that your loved one may withdraw and not feel like socializing. Sleep takes up more and more time. You may find this difficult because it's as if your loved one is slipping away from you. It feels like a corner has been turned, and it's a painful transition. This is part of your grieving

Sources of additional help

Booklet: *Journey's End: A Guide to Understanding the Dying Process* by Deborah Sigrist, B.S.N., R.N., Rochester, New York, Genesee Region Home Care, 1995. To order: (716) 262-1900.

Books: *Dying Well: The Prospect for Growth at the End of Life* by Ira Byock, M.D., New York, Penguin, 1997. *Final Gifts: Understanding the Special Awarenesses, Needs, and Communications of the Dying* by Maggie Callanan and Patricia Kelley, New York, Simon & Schuster, 1993. *The Rights of the Dying* by David Kessler, New York, HarperCollins, 1997. *The Dying Time* by Joan Furman, M.S.N., R.N. and David McNabb, New York, Bell Tower, 1997.

Organization: National Hospice Organization, 1901 N. Moore St., Suite 901, Arlington, VA 22209, (703) 243-5900.

process and a time to reach for support.

■ *Be aware of the spiritual dimension of dying.* Sometimes we're so focused on physical and emotional changes that we overlook the spiritual dimension. But like a quiet, underground river, it has been active all along.

It is not unusual for the dying to speak in metaphors about impending death, say the authors of *Final Gifts*. They may speak in terms of travel or journey, expressing an urgency to "get going, get to the door, find the key." Although the messages vary in content, the underlying message is, "I must go forth," and has a tone of anticipation.

As death nears, you may feel swept up in the process, like an ocean wave that is heading for shore. As families and caregivers, we watch, we comfort, we wait, we pray. Dying persons want to know that their lives have had meaning and value. We can help reassure them that this is the case.

Take heart
As your loved one journeys toward death, your companionship is a true and timeless gift. And while it's not for the faint-hearted, hopefully you'll do more than just endure or survive the journey. With preparation and support, you'll be transformed by it. ■

Deborah Sigrist is a registered nurse on the Inpatient Hospice Unit of Genesee Region Home Care in Rochester, New York. She facilitates a bereavement group, does community presentations on death, dying, and bereavement, and has authored Journey's End: A Guide to Understanding the Dying Process *(see resource section).*

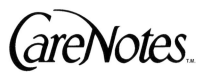

#21361

Abbey Press
St. Meinrad, IN 47577

This publication is recyclable and printed on recycled paper.

For a complete catalog of all of our caring publications,
call Toll-Free: 1-800-325-2511.

Address correspondence to:
One Caring Place, Abbey Press, St. Meinrad, IN 47577.

Cover photography by © Neena M. Mitchell - STOCK/ART IMAGES

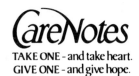

CareNotes

TAKE ONE - and take heart.
GIVE ONE - and give hope.

Saying Good-bye to a Loved One Who Is Dying

by Carol Luebering

Learning to wave "bye-bye" was one of our earliest accomplishments. Often we performed between screams, for watching loved ones walk away is a terrifying experience for tiny tots. Watching a loved one walk toward death's door sends the years of easy good-byes spinning away, and we are once again helpless, frightened, and inconsolable.

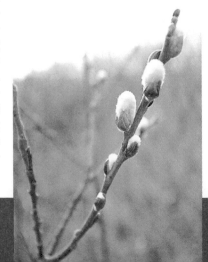

There is no easy way to say a last good-bye. If someone you love is dying, the weeks or months ahead hold much pain. But they also hold the makings of warm memories. I hope this Care-Note will help make your good-bye a graced experience.

Working your way through

My husband's mother spent the last six weeks of her life in a hospital bed in our dining room. Those six weeks were marked by stress and sorrow. Yet I also remember them as a season of such beauty that I now understand why Shakespeare's Juliet spoke of parting as a "sweet sorrow." Here are some suggestions to help you discover the beauty hidden within the pain.

■ **Be honest**. Don't play games about the seriousness of the illness. More than 20 years ago, a young doctor named Elisabeth Kubler-Ross set out to interview some dying patients—even though the hospital staff assured her that there were none in their institution! She quickly discovered that the dying indeed know their future, and are isolated by everyone else's refusal to discuss death's imminence.

How do you break through that isolation? My mother-in-law took the first step herself. When hope for her recovery failed, I hit the hospital at all kinds of odd hours, hoping to catch her without other visitors. When at last I succeeded, the first thing Mom said was, "I've wanted to talk to you alone. Does everyone know how sick I am?"

Let feelings into the conversation—your own and your loved one's. Talk about your fears about the course of the illness, your worries about the future, the grief you experience. And accept as normal whatever anger either one of you feels, whether it is directed at the unfairness of it all, at one of you—even at God.

Your openness will serve not only yourself, but also the dying person. Anything you feel—sorrow, anxiety, anger, fear—the dying feel much more. However great the loss you face, they are facing a greater one. A dying friend once taught me that.

Kay and I had spent an hour or more reminiscing about the many good times we'd had with our circle of friends. Suddenly Kay grew serious. "You know," she said, "I'm not afraid of dying. It's just that you know what you have here, and it's hard to leave." And I realized that even as I struggled to say good-bye to Kay, she was saying good-bye to everyone and everything she cared about.

People sometimes try to protect themselves from pain by shunning the dying. The more obviously mortal an illness becomes, the fewer visitors show up at the door. Even the closest people may distance themselves in other ways.

I started talking. I told him about my visit with Lisa and the new baby. And I talked about our other grandchildren. How dear they all were to us. How well they were developing....I talked about our courtship and the long years of waiting before we could get married and how young we had been. I talked about the farm and the good times we had there.

I talked for hours. Talked about the silly things, the good things, the times that I had cherished, about everything that had been important to me in our life together. I held his hand and poured my heart out. I told him over and over again how much I loved him and how happy he had always made me.

—Dr. Joyce Brothers, describing her last hours with her husband in *Widowed*

I watched our extended family around Mom's hospital bed after the surgery which erased the last hope of her recovery. All the people in the hospital room—myself included—were talking *over* Mom's bed: talking to each other, looking at each other. In the center Mom lay alone and abandoned in spite of all the company.

> *"For everything there is a season...a time to be born, and a time to die."*
>
> —Ecclesiastes 3:1-2

Backing off that way may seem to make the last good-bye easier, but it really doesn't. It only postpones the pain—and adds to it a lot of regrets. The end of a life is too precious to waste.

■ *Make good memories.* In the long run, memories are the only thing those who linger in this world get to keep. I can't prove it, but I suspect that memories are the only thing we get to take with us into the next world as well. The concept of life after death surely means that the love we have here is of enduring value, precious enough to preserve for eternity.

The dying cling to their memories. Unfinished business haunts them; they yearn to wrap things up and to know that their life really mattered. Give the one you love a hand.

One of the sweeter memories I cherish is taking my frail mother-in-law back to her apartment to gather up some things that were precious to her—sentimental possessions she wanted to give away while the pleasure was still hers: her father's pocket watch for the first grandson, a bit of wedding silver for the oldest granddaughter, an old pin for a daughter. I won't say it was an easy day. It wasn't. But I treasure the vase she gave me that day.

Most of us have more serious business pending than a few sentimental belongings: soured relationships and unuttered apologies. A friend wasn't sure she wanted to journey to her mother's bedside when the death sentence was pronounced. (This woman was not the stuff of Mother's Day cards.)

"This is your last chance to make good memories," my friend's husband wisely told her. And good memories are what she came home with—memories of a woman she could for the first time see as vulnerable, good memories of forgiveness extended and accepted, precious memories of good-bye as the first word well spoken between mother and daughter.

Help the person you love find assurance that his or her life has mattered—and, in the process, bring to the front of your mind the memories you yourself will keep. Get out the scrapbooks and photo albums and reminisce with the dying person. Invite other friends and family members to bring their memorabilia.

Call on business and volunteer associates for their fund of memories. My friend Kay found peace when the mayor of our town, spurred by the phone call

I no longer fear death, for as I held Jamie in my arms as she died, I saw nothing to fear. I no longer believe that death is an end.

—A bereaved mother, quoted by Elisabeth Kubler-Ross in *To Live Until We Say Good-bye* of another friend, presented a proclamation honoring her for her many years of volunteer work. My dying father and an old friend recalled making bathtub gin during Prohibition: rolling the jug back and forth between them to mix the ingredients and "to age it a little"—providing me with great amusement and a glimpse into an era before my time.

Plan a simple party, even if you have to hold it in a hospital room. A picture of Mom cutting a fancy cake has a place of honor on the wall in my family room. The whole family celebrated her 55th wedding anniversary—which fell just a couple of weeks before her death—with a simple religious service and a light lunch.

■ *Seek support.* There's a strange scene in the Old Testament (Exodus 17:8-13) where the Hebrews are engaged in battle. As long as Moses keeps his hands raised, the battle goes well for them; when they drop, the tide turns. So his friends come to his side and hold his arms up!

Isn't that what friends are for? When people ask you to tell them what they can do, they express genuine willingness; tell them what you need. Ask first for their shoulder and their ear—you'll need that kind of support long after death arrives. When you grow weary, ask for practical help with the laundry or the errands; let someone provide a meal or relieve you from caring for an invalid for an afternoon.

Your doctor or hospital social worker can direct

Sources of additional help

Books: *Someone You Love Is Dying* by Martin Shepard, M.D., New York, New York, Harmony, 1975. *Praying Our Goodbyes* by Joyce Rupp, Notre Dame, Indiana, Ave Maria, 1983.

Videotapes: *Ordinary People; Steel Magnolias.*

you to more skilled help from such organizations as Make Today Count, Hospice, or Cancer Care. Also, ask the doctor what to expect. No physician can predict the moment of death—that's in God's hands—but most can predict the likely course of an illness.

Take heart Good-byes are tough, no question. But a thought that helped me through my kids' teen years has also helped me through my good-byes: Some things can be held tightly only with open hands—a fragile butterfly, fresh-running water, love.

A dying person *will* slip from your grip no matter how tightly you cling. Hold your hands open wide enough to receive a treasury of stored memories, the support of friends and strangers, the love and honesty you want in your relationship to the end.

And know that your hands are held gently by someone who never grips too tightly and yet never lets go. The God who gave us life and love will never let it go to waste. ■

Carol Luebering is a free-lance writer and a book and homily service editor with St. Anthony Messenger Press. Her works include the CareNotes Planning the Funeral of Someone You Love, Getting Through the Annual Reminders of Your Loss, *and* Helping a Child Grieve and Grow.

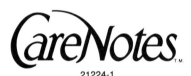

21224-1

Abbey Press
St. Meinrad, IN 47577

50-21224-1. This publication is recyclable and printed on recycled paper.

For a complete catalog of all of our caring publications,
call Toll-Free: 1-800-325-2511.

Address correspondence to:
One Caring Place, Abbey Press, St. Meinrad, IN 47577.

Cover photograph by Neena M. Wilmot-STOCK/ART IMAGES